THE EA AFTER 50

The Ultimate Weight Loss Recipes for People Over 50 to Lose Fats and Live Healthy

Amelia McDermott

Copyright © 2019 by Amelia McDermott - All rights reserved.

All other copyrights & trademarks are the properties of their respective owners; Reproduction of any part of this book without the permission of the copyright owners is illegal-except with the inclusion of brief quotes in a review of the work

Contents

How To Start A keto Diet When You're Over 50?........1

List of Foods On The Keto Diet. 3

How Does Aging Affect Your Nutritional Needs? 6

Foods and diets to avoid. 22

Breakfast Recipes for After 50: 25

    Taco Egg Muffins..25

    Deviled eggs 27

Tasty Coconut Almond Porridge 28

Delicious Keto Cereal with Berries 30

    Spinach and Red pepper Frittata. 31

Tasty Chocolate Chia Pudding with Almonds.............34

Heavenly Parsley Quiche..35

Mouthwatering Hot Oatmeal 37

Yummy Vanilla Turmeric Oatmeal 38

    Coconut Porridge 39

    Crust less Quiche Lorraine. 40

Simple Tasty Keto Tortillas...41

Almond Hemp Oatmeal 43

Delicious Keto Muesli...44

Cappuccino Soft Cheese 46

Lunch Recipes for After 50: 46

    Cream Cheese Stuffed Baby Peppers. 46

    Artichoke Dip 48

Avocado Tuna Melt Bites 49

    Taco meat. 58

    Green Beans with Bacon. 70

    Yummy Eggplant Burgers 72

Greek Chicken Salad 75

Cranberry Walnut Salad 75

Watermelon, Mint & Feta Salad 77

Pork Tenderloin 77

    Beef And Broccoli. 79

    Snacks And Sides for After 50: 81

    Asparagus Fries. 81

    Kale chips. 83

Chocó Roasted Almonds 84

Cheese Crackers 85

Peanut Butter Smoothie 86

Salami Cheese Roll-ups 87

Keto Chocolate Pudding 88

Blueberry Mug Cake 89

    Guacamole 91

    Zucchini Noodles 92

    Cauliflower Soufflé. 93

Strawberry Avocado Mousse 94

Egg Mayo 95

Green Smoothie 96

Almond Butter Fudge 97

Chocolate Hazelnut Smoothie 98

Aztec Chocolate Smoothie 98

Blackberry Coconut Fat Bombs 99

Strawberry Protein Smoothie 100

Almond Butter Balls 101

Berry Protein Smoothie 102

Cheddar Muffin 103

Keto Jelly 105

    Dinner Recipes for After 50: 106

    Whole Chicken 106

    Lamb Shanks: 107

Mushroom Stake 109

Keto Avocado Sushi 111

Romaine Saltimbocca Chicken 112

Stake & ghee Broccoli 113

Keto Hot Salami Pizza 114

Superfood Soup with Air Cured Beef 116

Ham & Cheese Pizza with Asparagus 117

Stake & Marinated Zucchini 118

Baked Trout Fillets with Sour Cream & Broccoli 119

Pizza Chicken Skillet 120

    Jamaican Jerk Pork Roast 122

    Zuppa Toscana 124

    Thai Shrimp Soup. 125

Dessert: 127

    Chocolate Avocado Ice Cream 127

    Mocha Mouse. 129

    Strawberry Rhubarb Custard 130

    Crème Brulee 132

    Pumpkin Pie Pudding. 134

How To Start A keto Diet When You're Over 50?

When you are over 50 and trying to lose weight, the diet options available are dizzying! Every magazine has a different "magic" formula for weight loss and it can be difficult to find a plan that works for you.

The combination of changing hormone levels and loss of muscle mass can make it more difficult for women over 50 to lose weight. While keto diet is a popular weight loss tool, it comes with some other health benefits, including knee pain reduction, according to a 2019 study published in the journal medicine. However, before you ditch all your bread and pasta, ensure you:

1. **Increase your intake of high-quality fats**: Aim to get at least 70% of your calories from healthy fats, such as avocado oil, extra virgin, coconut oil, olive

oil, nuts, avocado, fatty fish like salmon, meats, nut butter eggs.

2. **Try a short- term fat-fast**. A short-term, high-fat fast- Such as an egg fast, can help into ketosis faster, as its very low in carbs and high in fat,

3. **Eat 20-50 grams of carbs per day**. This should encourage your body to produce ketones. People who struggle to enter ketosis may need to stick to the lower end of the scale.

4. **Track your carb intak**e: This helps to ensure you to eat 20- 50 grams of carbs per day and don't underestimate your carb intake.

5. **Avoid eating out**: while there are many keto friendly resultants eating out makes it harder to track your crabs.

6. **Try intermittent fasting**: fasts like intermittent fasting may help your body shift its fuel source from carbs to fat while maintaining its energy balance.

7. **Be aware of hidden carb sources**: it's easy to overlook condiments, but many sources and dressings are high in carbs.
8. **Exercise more.** Physical activity can deplete your body's glycogen stores, which encourages your liver to increase its production of ketosis. Studies show that working out in a fasted state can help increase ketone levels.
9. **Test your ketone levels regularly**: testing ketone levels helps give you an idea of whether you're in ketosis which lets you adjust your diet accordingly.
10. **Use a medium chain** triglyceride (MCT) supplement. MCTs are a type of fat that's rapidly absorbed by your body easily converted into ketosis.

List of Foods On The Keto Diet.

1. Seaford. Such as fish and shellfish. Examples of shellfish are: crabs, shrimps, langoustine, lobster, prawns, crayfish, krill, and barnacles. Fish such as cod, salmon,

trout, tuna, haddock, sea bream, plaice and shark.
2. Low carb vegetables. Vegetables are nutritious and versatile and help to reduce the risk of disease. Such as, bell pepper, Broccoli, asparagus, Mushrooms, spinach, avocados, green beans, lettuce, carrots, garlic, cucumbers, tomatoes, cabbage, onions, Egg plant, zucchini, kale Radishes, artichokes, cauliflower, Carley, and brussels sprouts.
3. Cheese. Eating cheese regularly help reduce the loss of muscle mass and strength that occurs with aging.
4. Avocados. Help improve cholesterol and triglyceride levels.
5. Meat and poultry. Fresh meat and poultry contain no Carbs, are rich in B vitamins and several minerals.
6. Egg. Egg trigger hormones that increase feelings of fullness and keep blood sugar levels stable.

7. Coconut oil. It's helps to increase ketone production and promote the loss of weight, belly fat and obese adult.
8. Plain greek yogurt and cottage cheese. Help decrease appetite and promote feelings of fullness.
9. Olive oil. It's protect heart healthy by decreasing inflammation and improving artery function.
10. Nuts and seeds. Such as. Cashew: eight grams net carbs (nine)grams of total carbs, Almonds: three grams net carbs (six grams of total carbs). Brazil nuts : one gram net carbs ((three grams total carbs). Macadamia nuts : two grams net carbs (four grams total carbs). Walnuts : two grams net carbs (four grams total carbs). Pumpkin seeds : four grams net carbs (five grams total carbs). Are heart healthy high in fiber and at least to healthier aging.

11. Berries. Are low in carbs and high in fiber. Such as, Blackberries: Five grams net carbs (ten grams total carbs). Blueberries : twelve grams net carbs (fourteen grams of total carbs). Raspberries: six grams net carbs (twelve grams total carbs). Strawberries: six grams net carbs (eight grams total carbs).
12. Olives: it helps to prevent bone loss and decrease blood pressure.
13. Unsweetened coffee and Tea. Are healthy carb free drinks, it helps boost your metabolic rate as well physical and mental performance. They can also reduce your risk of diabetes.
14. Dark chocolate and cocoa powder. Help reduce the risk of heart disease and contain 3-10 grams of net carbs.

How Does Aging Affect Your Nutritional Needs?

Eating healthy becomes especially important as you age. That's because aging is linked to a variety of changes, including nutrient deficiencies, decreased quality of life and poor health outcomes.

Luckily, there are things you can do to help prevent deficiencies and other age-related changes. For example, eating nutrient-rich foods and taking the appropriate supplements can help keep you healthy as you age.

This guide explains how your nutritional needs change as you age, including how to address them.

Aging is linked to a variety of changes in the body, including muscle loss, thinner skin and less stomach acid.

Some of these changes can make you prone to nutrient deficiencies, while others can affect your senses and quality of life.

For example, studies have estimated that 20% of elderly people have atrophic gastritis, a condition in which chronic inflammation has damaged the cells that produce stomach acid

Low stomach acid can affect the absorption of nutrients, such as vitamin B12, calcium, iron and magnesium.

Another challenge of aging is a reduced need for calories. Unfortunately, this creates a nutritional dilemma. Older adults need to get just as much, if not more, of some nutrients, all while eating fewer calories.

Fortunately, eating a variety of whole foods and taking a supplement can help you meet your nutrient needs.

Another issue people may experience as they age is a reduction in their body's ability to recognize vital senses like hunger and thirst.

This could make you prone to dehydration and unintentional weight loss. And the older you get, the harsher these consequences may be.

Needing Fewer Calories, but More Nutrients

A person's daily calorie needs depend on their height, weight, muscle mass, activity level and several other factors.

Older adults may need fewer calories to maintain their weight, since they tend to move and exercise less and carry less muscle

If you continue to eat the same number of calories per day as you did when you were younger, you could easily gain extra fat, especially around the belly area.

This is especially true in postmenopausal women, as the decline in estrogen levels seen during this time may promote belly fat storage.

However, even though older adults need fewer calories, they need just as high or even higher levels of some nutrients, compared to younger people.

This makes it very important for older people to eat a variety of whole foods, such as fruits, vegetables, fish and lean meats. These healthy staples can help you fight nutrient deficiencies, without expanding your waistline.

Nutrients that become especially important as you age include protein, vitamin D, calcium and vitamin B12.

You Can Benefit From More Protein

It's common to lose muscle and strength as you age. In fact, the average adult loses 3–8% of their muscle mass each decade after age 30 (8Trusted Source).

This loss of muscle mass and strength is known as sarcopenia. It's a major cause of weakness, fractures and poor health among the elderly.

Eating more protein can help your body maintain muscle and fight sarcopenia. One study followed 2,066 elderly people over three years. It found those who ate the most protein daily lost 40% less muscle mass than people who ate the least. Also, a review of 20 recent studies in elderly people found that eating more protein or taking protein supplements may slow the rate of muscle loss, increase muscle mass and help build more muscle.

Furthermore, combining a protein-rich diet with resistance exercise seems to be the most effective way to fight sarcopenia. You can find many simple ways to increase your protein intake here.

You May Benefit From More Fiber

Constipation is a common health problem among the elderly. It's especially common in people over 65, and it's two to three times more common in women.

That's because people at this age tend to move less and be more likely to take medications that have constipation as a side effect.

Eating fiber may help relieve constipation. It passes through the gut undigested, helping form stool and promote regular bowel movements.

In an analysis of five studies, scientists found that dietary fiber helped stimulate bowel movements in people with constipation.

Additionally, a high-fiber diet may prevent diverticular disease, a condition in which small pouches form along the colon wall and become infected or inflamed. This condition is especially common among the elderly.

Diverticular disease is often viewed as a disease of the Western diet. It's incredibly common, affecting up to 50% of people over age 50 in Western countries.

Conversely, diverticular disease is almost absent in populations with higher fiber intakes. For example, in Japan and Africa, diverticular disease affects less than 0.2% of people.

SUMMARY:
Bowel-related issues, including constipation and diverticular disease, can occur as you age. You can help protect yourself by increasing your fiber intake.

You Need More Calcium and Vitamin D
Calcium and vitamin D are two of the most important nutrients for bone health. Calcium

helps build and maintain healthy bones; while vitamin D helps the body absorbs calcium.

Unfortunately, older adults tend to absorb less calcium from their diets. Human and animal studies have found that the gut tends to absorb less calcium with age.

However, the reduction in calcium absorption is likely caused by a vitamin D deficiency, since aging can make the body less efficient at producing it.

Your body can make vitamin D from the cholesterol in your skin when it is exposed to sunlight. However, aging can make the skin thinner, which reduces its ability to make vitamin D.

Together, these changes could prevent you from getting enough calcium and vitamin D, promoting bone loss and increasing your risk of fractures.

To counter aging's effects on your vitamin D and calcium levels, it's necessary to consume more calcium and vitamin D through foods and supplements.

A variety of foods contain calcium, including dairy products and dark green, leafy vegetables. You can find other great sources of calcium here.

Meanwhile, vitamin D is found in a variety of fish, such as salmon and herring. You can find other great sources of vitamin D here.

Older people can also benefit from taking a vitamin D supplement like cod liver oil.

SUMMARY:

Calcium and vitamin D are important nutrients for maintaining optimal bone health. Your body stands to benefit from getting more calcium and vitamin D as you age.

You May Need More Vitamin B12

Vitamin B12 is a water-soluble vitamin also known as cobalamin. It's essential for making red blood cells and maintaining healthy brain function.

Unfortunately, studies estimate that 10-30% of people over age 50 have a reduced ability to absorb vitamin B12 from their diet. Over time, this could cause a vitamin B12 deficiency.

Vitamin B12 in the diet is bound to proteins in the food you eat. Before your body can use it, stomach acid must help it separate from these food proteins. Older people are more likely to have conditions that reduce stomach acid production, leading to less vitamin B12 absorption from food. Atrophic gastritis is one condition that can cause this

Additionally, older people who follow a vegan or vegetarian diet are less likely to eat rich sources of vitamin B12, since it's more abundant in animal foods such as eggs, fish, meat and dairy.

For this reason, older people can benefit from taking a vitamin B12 supplement or consuming foods fortified with vitamin B12.

These fortified foods contain crystalline vitamin B12, which is not bound to food proteins. So people who produce less than the normal amount of stomach acid can still absorb it.

SUMMARY:

Aging increases the risk of a vitamin B12 deficiency. Older adults can especially benefit from taking a vitamin B12 supplement or consuming foods fortified with vitamin B12.

Other Nutrients That May Help You as You Age

Several other nutrients may benefit you as you age, including:

Potassium: A higher potassium intake is associated with a lower risk of high blood pressure, kidney stones, osteoporosis and heart disease, all of which are more common among the elderly.

Omega-3 fatty acids: Heart disease is the leading cause of death among the elderly. Studies have shown that omega-3 fatty acids can lower heart disease risk factors like high blood pressure and triglycerides.

Magnesium: Magnesium is an important mineral in the body. Unfortunately, elderly people are at risk of deficiency because of poor intake, medication use and age-related changes in gut function.

Iron: Deficiency is common in elderly people. This may cause anemia, a condition in which the blood does not supply enough oxygen to the body.

Most of these nutrients can be obtained from a diet rich in fruits, vegetables, fish and lean meats. However, people who follow a vegetarian or vegan diet could benefit from taking an iron or omega-3 supplement.

Although iron is found in a variety of vegetables, plant sources of iron are not absorbed as well as meat sources of iron. Omega-3 fats are mostly found in fish.

SUMMARY:

Potassium, magnesium, omega-3 fatty acids and iron are other nutrients you can benefit from as you get older.

You Are More Prone to Dehydration

Water makes up about 60% of your body. It's important to stay hydrated at any age, since your body constantly loses water, mainly through sweat and urine.

Additionally, aging can make you prone to dehydration. Your body detects thirst through receptors found in the brain and throughout the body.

However, as you age, these receptors may become less sensitive to water changes, making it harder for them to detect thirst.

Additionally, your kidneys help your body conserve water, but they tend to lose function as you age.

Unfortunately, dehydration comes with harsh consequences for older people. Long-term dehydration can reduce the fluid in your cells, reducing your ability to absorb medicine, worsening medical conditions and increasing fatigue.

That's why it's important to make a conscious effort to drink enough water daily. If you find drinking water a challenge, try having one to two glasses of water with each meal. Otherwise, try carrying a water bottle as you go about your day.

SUMMARY:
Drinking an adequate amount of water is important as you age, as your body may become less able to recognize the signs of dehydration.

You May Struggle to Eat Enough Food

Another troubling concern for elderly people is decreased appetite. If this issue isn't addressed, it can lead to unintended weight loss and nutritional deficiencies. A loss of appetite is also linked to poor health and a higher risk of death.

Factors that could cause older adults to have a poor appetite include changes in hormones, taste and smell, as well as changes in life circumstances.

Studies have found that older people tend to have lower levels of hunger hormones and higher levels of fullness hormones, which means they could get hungry less often and feel fuller more quickly.

In a small study with 11 elderly people and 11 young adults, researchers found that elderly participants had significantly lower levels of the hunger hormone ghrelin before a meal.

Additionally, several studies have found that elderly people have higher levels of the fullness hormones cholecystokinin and leptin.

Aging can also affect your sense of smell and taste, making food seem less appealing. Other factors that may cause poor appetite include tooth loss, loneliness, underlying illness and medications that can decrease appetite

If you find it difficult to eat large meals, try dividing your meals into smaller portions and have them every few hours. Otherwise, try to establish a habit of eating healthy snacks like almonds, yogurt and boiled eggs, which provide lots of nutrients and a good number of calories.

SUMMARY:

It's common for elderly people to experience reduced appetite. If this issue isn't addressed, it can lead to weight loss, nutritional deficiencies and poor health.

The Bottom Line

Aging is linked to changes that can make you prone to deficiencies in calcium, vitamin D, vitamin B12, iron, magnesium and several other important nutrients.

It may also reduce your ability to recognize sensations like hunger and thirst. Luckily, you can take actions to prevent these deficiencies.

Make a conscious effort to stay on top of your water and food intake, eat a variety of nutrient-rich foods and consider taking a supplement. All these actions can help you fight deficiencies and stay healthy as you get older.

Foods and diets to avoid.

Sugar :

This is the big no-no. Cut out all soft drinks, fruit juice, sports drinks and "vitamin water" (these are all basically sugar water). Avoid sweets, candy, cakes, cookies, chocolate bars, donuts, frozen treats and breakfast cereals.

Read labels for hidden sugars, especially in sauces, condiments, drinks, dressings and packaged goods. Honey, maple syrup, and agave are also sugars. Ideally try to avoid or limit artificial sweeteners as well. Full keto sweeteners guide

Starch: Bread, pasta, rice, potatoes (including sweet potatoes), French fries, potato chips, porridge, muesli and so on. Avoid whole grain products as well.

Legumes, such as beans and lentils, are high in carbs too. Small amounts of certain root vegetables (other than potatoes and sweet potatoes) may be OK.

Note that there are many good potential replacements for these foods, that work on a keto diet. Here are a few of them:

- Keto breads
- Keto "pasta"
- Keto "rice"
- Keto porridge

Beer: Liquid bread. Full of rapidly absorbed carbs. But there are a few lower-carb beers

Fruit: Very sweet, lots of sugar. Eat once in a while perhaps. Treat fruit as a natural form of candy. Learn more

Also avoid

Margarine: It's industrially produced imitated butter with a very high content of omega-6 fat. It has no obvious health benefits, and many people feel that it tastes worse than butter. It might be linked to asthma, allergies and other inflammatory diseases, possibly because of the high omega-6 content.

Beware!

The ketogenic diet has recently become very popular, and many food companies want to cash in by putting a "ketogenic" or "low carb" label on a new product. Be very cautious of special "keto" or "low-carb" products, such as pastas, chocolate bars, energy bars, protein powders, snack foods, cakes, cookies and other "low carb" or "ketogenic" treats. Read all labels carefully for natural low carb ingredients. The fewer ingredients the better.

These packaged products generally do not work well for weight loss and for correcting metabolic issues. They may have hidden carbs not declared on the label, or they may keep you attached to cravings and even addictions to the high-carb foods they attempt to replace.

Often you will see that a product is full of additives, sugar alcohols and other sweeteners. They are often in essence an ultra-processed junk food with a "keto" label." And the labels may even lie. For example, a few years ago a large pasta company was fined $8 million for lying about the carb content of their products.

Don't replace high-carb junk with keto junk. If you want a treat, make a low-carb version of a dessert or treat yourself, using our dessert or treat guide. You will likely have more life-long success on the keto diet if you adapt your palate so that you no longer want, need, or crave these sorts of foods.

Beware of labels that say "net carbs". That might sometimes be a form of creative marketing to hide the true carb content.

Breakfast Recipes for After 50:

Taco Egg Muffins

Nutritional Info:

Calories: 330

Fat: 17g

Protein: 21g

Net Carbs: 69

Ingredients:

- 8 oz. ground beef
- 3 tbsp. Taco Seasoning (get the recipe here)
- 2 oz. onion, diced
- 12 large eggs
- 1 cup sharp cheddar cheese, shredded
- 3 oz. mixed bell peppers, diced
- 10 black olives, sliced
- ½ cup sour cream
- ½ cup salsa

Directions:

1. Preheat oven to 350° lightly oil a muffin tin. Or you can use a non-stick silicone bakeware. In a large skillet over medium-high heat, add ground beef and onions. Sauté until ground beef is browned. Drain

excess grease from the pan. Mix in 1/3 cup water and taco seasoning. Reduce heat to low and allow to simmer 3-4 minutes until thickened.
2. In a large mixing bowl, fork whisk eggs. Mix in cheese, bell peppers, and olives.
3. Mix meat into egg mixture. Pour mixture into muffin tin. This should fill 12 spots. Bake for 25 minutes.
4. Top each muffin with sour cream and salsa prior to serving.

Deviled eggs

Nutrition Facts:

Calories; 327

Fat; 26

Carbohydrates; 4.7 g

Protein; 19.3g

Cholesterol; 563 mg

Sodium; 902 mg

Ingredients:

- 6 hard-cooked eggs
- 2 tablespoons mayonnaise
- 1 teaspoon white sugar
- 1 teaspoon white vinegar
- 1 teaspoon prepared mustard
- 1/2 teaspoon salt.
- 1 tablespoon finely chopped onion.
- 1 tablespoon finely chopped celery.
- 1 pinch paprika, or to taste.

Directions:

1. Slice eggs in half lengthwise and remove yolks; set whites aside.
2. Mash yolks with a fork in a small bowl.
3. Stir in mayonnaise, sugar, vinegar, mustard, salt, onion, and celery; mix well. Stuff or pipe egg yolk mixture into egg whites.
4. Sprinkle with paprika. Refrigerate until serving.

Tasty Coconut Almond Porridge

Nutrition Info.

Total calories: 739
Calories from fat: 492
Total fat: 58.7g
Saturated fat: 30.7g
Total Carbohydrates: 35.5g
Fiber: 8.0g
Net carbohydrates: 27.5g
Protein: 19.0g

Ingredients:
- Half (½) cup shredded coconut
- Two (2) tbsp. ground almonds or almond flour
- Three quarter (3/4) cup almond milk
- Half (½) cup coconut milk
- One (1) egg yolk
- One quarter (1/4) cup slivered almonds

Directions:
1. In a small pot, add the coconut, almonds, and almond milk. Bring to a simmer and cook for five minutes, adding more water if needed.
2. Use a fork to whisk the egg yolk and the coconut cream and add.

3. Gently cook until the porridge thickens
4. Topped with slivered almonds and serve.

Delicious Keto Cereal with Berries

Nutrition Info.
Total calories: 625
Calories from fat: 500
Total fat: 59.0g
Saturated fat: 23.3g
Total carbohydrates: 23.3g
Fiber: 11.2g
Net carbohydrates: 12.1g
Protein: 10.0g

Ingredients:
- One quarter (1/4) cup toasted coconut flakes
- One quarter (1/4) cup slivered almonds
- Two (2) tbsp. chopped hazelnuts
- Half (½) cup half and half
- Half (½) cup berries

Directions:
1. In a bowl, stir together the coconut,

almonds, and hazelnuts.

2. Pour the half and half over and top with berries. Enjoy!

Spinach and Red pepper Frittata.

Ingredients:

- 6-ounce bag baby spinach, or 1 bunch spinach, washed and stemmed
- tablespoons extra virgin olive oil
- red bell peppers, seeded and cut in small dice
- 1 to 2 garlic cloves (to taste), minced
- 10 fresh marjoram leaves, chopped
- Salt
- 8 eggs
- Freshly ground pepper
- 2 tablespoons low-fat milk

Directions:

1. Steam spinach above an inch boiling water until just wilted, about two minutes; or wilt in a large frying pan with the water left on the leaves after washing. Remove from the

heat, rinse with cold water and squeeze out excess water. Chop fine, and set aside.

2. Heat 1 tablespoon of the olive oil over medium heat in a heavy 10-inch nonstick skillet. Add the bell peppers. Cook, stirring often, until tender, five to eight minutes. Add garlic and salt to taste, stir for about half a minute, and stir in the chopped spinach and marjoram. Stir together for a few seconds, then remove from the heat and set aside.

3. Beat the eggs in a large bowl. Stir in the salt (about 1/2 teaspoon), pepper, milk, spinach and red peppers. Clean and dry the pan, and return to the burner, set on medium-high. Heat the remaining tablespoon of olive oil in the skillet. Drop a bit of egg into the pan; if it sizzles and cooks at once, the pan is ready. Pour in the egg mixture. Tilt the pan to distribute the eggs and filling evenly over the surface. Shake the pan gently, tilting it

slightly with one hand while lifting up the edges of the frittata with a spatula in your other hand, to let the eggs run underneath during the first few minutes of cooking.

4. Turn the heat to low, cover and cook 10 minutes, shaking the pan gently every once in a while. From time to time, remove the lid, tilt the pan, and loosen the bottom of the frittata with a wooden spatula so that it doesn't burn. The bottom should turn a golden color. The eggs should be just about set; cook a few minutes longer if they're not.

5. Meanwhile, heat the broiler. Uncover the pan and place under the broiler, not too close to the heat, for one to three minutes, watching very carefully to make sure the top doesn't burn (at most, it should brown very slightly and puff under the broiler). Remove from the heat, shake the pan to make sure the frittata isn't sticking, and allow it to cool for at least five minutes and

for as long as 15 minutes. Loosen the edges with a wooden or plastic spatula. Carefully slide from the pan onto a large round platter. Cut into wedges or into smaller bite-size diamonds.
6. Serve hot, warm, at room temperature or cold.

Tasty Chocolate Chia Pudding with Almonds

Nutrition Info.
Total calories: 577
Calories from fat: 465
Total fat: 54.5g
Saturated fat: 29.7g
Total carbohydrates: 20.6g
Fiber: 14.2g
Net carbohydrates: 6.4g
Protein: 10.6g

Ingredients:
- Three (3) tbsp. chia seeds
- One quarter (1/4) cup heavy cream
- Three quarter (3/4) cup water
- One (1) tbsp. MCT oil

- One (1) tbsp. cocoa powder
- Sweetener, optional
- Two (2) tbsp. slivered almonds

Directions:
1. Combine the first six ingredients and allow to sit for eight-twelve hours, shaking occasionally. Served with slivered almonds.

Heavenly Parsley Quiche

Nutrition Info.
Total carbs: 3.8g
Net carbs: 3g
Protein 19.4 g
Fat: 33.9g
Calories- per serving, 3 mini quiches: 402

Ingredients:
- Half (½) tbsp. ghee
- Two (2) tbsp. broccoli, diced
- Half (½) tbsp. freshly chopped parsley
- Two (2) medium eggs

- One (1) tbsp. parmesan cheese, shredded
- One (1) pinch of salt
- One (1) pinch of sweet paprika
- Two (2) tbsp. heavy whipping cream
- One (1) tbsp. grated Swiss cheese

Instructions:

1. Preheat your oven to 175 degrees F. dice your broccoli and the grated cheese.
2. Whisk the eggs with parmesan, salt, paprika, and cream.
3. Coat three small cup muffin tins with ghee. Scatter broccoli and parsley over the bottom of each cup. Distribute the egg mixture into the cups evenly.
4. Use the grated Swiss cheese to top each. Bake until the quiches are browned and puffed on top, for twenty-thirty minutes, rotating the tray halfway through.
5. Allow to cool off for a few minutes. Eat instantly or store in the refrigerator for up to four days.

Mouthwatering Hot Oatmeal

Nutrition Info
Calories: 120
Total carbs: 7g
Fat: 10g
Net carbs: 2g
Protein: 3g

Ingredients:
- Two (2) tbsp. unsweetened coconut flakes
- Half (½) cup unsweetened almond milk or coconut milk
- Three (¾) tbsp. coconut flour
- Three (¾) tbsp. flaxseed meal
- One (1) sprinkle vanilla extract
- One (1) teaspoon stevia

Instructions:
1. Use the medium pot to toast the coconut flakes over medium heat until golden. Stir frequently to avoid burning.
2. Stir in the almond milk or coconut milk and water. Cover and bring to boil.

3. Once the boiling point is reached, remove from heat and add the remaining ingredients.

Yummy Vanilla Turmeric Oatmeal

Nutrition Info:
Calories: 310
Fat: 27g
Total carbs: 6g
Net carbs: 3g
Protein: 11g

Ingredients:
- Three (3) tbsp. hemp hearts
- One quarter (1/4) cup coconut milk
- One (1) tsp. Chia seeds
- Half (½) tsp. turmeric powder
- Half (½) tsp. vanilla extract
- Two (2) drops of stevia

Instructions:
1. Combine all ingredients in a bowl and mix thoroughly.
2. Place in the fridge overnight, or a

minimum of four hours.

Coconut Porridge

Nutrition Info:

Net Carbs; 6g

Total Carbs; 21g

15g Fiber; 15g

Fat, 279

Protein, 15g

Ingredients:

- ¾ cup of Water
- 1/8 teaspoon of Kosher Salt
- 1 large Egg
- 2 teaspoon of Butter
- 1 tablespoon of Coconut Milk
- 2 tablespoons of Flax Seeds
- ½ cup of Blueberries
- 2 tbsp. of Coconut Flour by Native

Directions:

1. Place ground flax seeds, coconut flour, water and salt in a small saucepan. Heat

mixture on medium-high heat until slightly thickened.
2. Beat an egg. Take mixer off the heat, add half of the egg, whisk. Then add the rest of the egg. Whisk mixture until thickened and egg is cooked through.
3. Remove from the heat, stir in butter. Top porridge with coconut milk and blueberries, if desired.

Crust less Quiche Lorraine.

Nutrition Info:

Calories; 309

Fat; 23.7g

Carbohydrates; 4.89

Protein; 20.4g

Cholesterol; 209 mg

Sodium; 546 mg

Ingredients:

- 1 tablespoon vegetable oil
- 1 onion, chopped
- 1 (10 ounce) package frozen chopped spinach, thawed and drained

- 5 eggs, beaten
- 3 cups shredded Muenster cheese
- 1/4 teaspoon salt
- 1/8 teaspoon ground black pepper.

Directions:

1. Preheat oven to 350 degrees F (175 degrees C). Lightly grease a 9 inch pie pan.
2. Heat the oil in a large skillet over medium-high heat. Add onions and cook, stirring occasionally, until onions are soft. Stir in spinach and continue cooking until excess moisture has evaporated.
3. In a large bowl, combine eggs, cheese, salt and pepper. Add spinach mixture and stir to blend. Scoop into prepared pie pan.
4. Bake in preheated oven until eggs have set, about 30 minutes. Let cool for 10 minutes before serving.

Simple Tasty Keto Tortillas

Nutrition Info.

Calories for 2 tortillas: 140
Fat: 12.09g
Total carbs: 3g
Net carbs: 1.37g
Protein: 4.37g

Ingredients:
- One (1) large egg white
- Two (2) tbsp. coconut flour
- One (1) tsp. water
- One (1) sprinkle baking powder
- One (1) small pinch of salt
- One (1) pinch of garlic powder
- One (1) pinch of onion powder
- One (1) pinch of chili powder

Instructions:
1. In a bowl, add egg white, baking powder, coconut flour, and water. Combine very well and let it be a uniform watery mixture.
2. You can add seasonings (optional).
3. Heat any desirable size of the skillet to low heat. When the pan is hot, use the cooking

spray to spray it, and drop some of the mixtures into the center.
4. As fast as possible, tilt the skillet on all edge to spread the batter as thin as possible. In the areas not covered, you can always add more.
5. Let it cook for two minutes until it starts to bubble, or you lift it up, and the other side has browned.
6. Flip and cook for extra one minute.
7. Repeat the process for a second tortilla. Lay the two tortillas on some kitchen paper to absorb the oil.
8. Use two tbsp. of unsalted butter to spread on it. Enjoy!

Almond Hemp Oatmeal

Nutrition Info.
Calories: 310
Fat: 27g
Total carbs: 6g
Net carbs: 3
Protein: 11g

Ingredients:
- Three (3) tbsp. hemp hearts
- One quarter (1/4) cup coconut milk
- One (1) tsp. chopped, almonds
- One (1) tsp. dark chocolate chips
- One (1) tsp. shredded coconut
- One (1) pinch vanilla extract
- One (1) pinch natural Stevia

Instructions:
1. Combine all the ingredients in a bowl and mix very well.
2. Place in the fridge overnight, or a minimum of four hours

Delicious Keto Muesli

Nutrition Info.
Calories: 441.36
Fat: 45.8g
Total carbs: 6.1g
Net carbs: 2.8g
Protein: 6.9g

Ingredients:
- One (1) tbsp. sunflower seeds
- One (1) tbsp. unsweetened flaked coconut
- One (1) tbsp. pumpkin seeds
- One (1) tbsp. sliced almonds
- One (1) tsp. pecans, grinded
- Two (2) tbsp. coconut oil
- One (1) tsp. hemp hearts
- One (1) pinch of each: vanilla extract, and cinnamon
- One (1) tsp. natural, Stevia
- Two (2) tbsp. of ghee

Instructions:
1. Take a large bowl and stir together all ingredients until well combined.
2. Pour on a rimmed baking pan and bake at 180 degrees F. for about seven-eight minutes.
3. Let it cool off. Serve with almond milk, and it can be stored in an airtight container.

Cappuccino Soft Cheese

Nutrition Info
Calories: 412.85
Fat: 41.4g
Total carbs: 3.46g
Net carbs: 3.46
Protein: 3.57g

Ingredients:

- Half (½) cup lactose-free mascarpone cheese
- One (1) tsp. natural Stevia powder
- One (1) tsp. vanilla extract
- One (1) tbsp. instant coffee powder

Instructions:

1. Use a food mixer to blend all ingredients until creamy. In the summer season, it can be mixed with ice.

     Lunch Recipes for After 50:

Cream Cheese Stuffed Baby Peppers.

Nutrition Info:

Calories 114

Fat 10g 15%

Saturated Fat 4g 25%

Cholesterol 23mg 8%

Sodium 91mg 4%

Potassium 132mg 4%

Carbohydrates 4g 1%

Fiber 1g 4%

Sugar 2g 2%

Protein 4g 8%

Ingredients:
- 12 ounces baby bell peppers
- 4 ounces cream cheese room temperature, reduced fat or regular
- 2 ounces cheddar cheese shredded
- 1/2 small jalapeno minced (about 1 tablespoon)
- 1/4 cup walnuts chopped (about 1 ounce)

Directions:
1. Preheat the oven to 400°F. Line a baking sheet with foil or parchment paper for easier cleanup, if desired.

2. Slice the bell peppers in half lengthwise and discard seeds & ribs. Set aside.
3. In a medium bowl, stir together cream cheese, cheddar cheese, walnuts and jalapeño until combined.
4. Spoon mixture into the bell pepper halves and transfer to the baking sheet. Repeat with all the bell peppers. Bake for 15-25 minutes depending on how browned you want the cheese.
5. Serve hot or room temperature. Enjoy!

Artichoke Dip

Nutrition Info:

Calories; 221

Fat; 19.2g

Carbohydrates; 6.69

Protein; 6.4g
Cholesterol; 23 mg

Sodium; 481 mg

Ingredients:

- 1/2 cup mayonnaise

- 1/2 cup sour cream
- 1 cup grated Parmesan cheese 1 (14 ounce) can artichoke hearts, drained
- 1/2 cup minced red onion
- 1 tablespoon of lemon juice, salt and pepper to taste.

Directions:

1. Preheat oven to 400 degrees F (200 degrees C).
2. In a medium-sized mixing bowl, stir together mayonnaise, sour cream, Parmesan cheese and onion. When these ingredients are combined, mix in artichoke hearts, lemon juice, salt and pepper. Transfer mixture to a shallow baking dish.
3. Bake at 400 degrees F (200 degrees C) for 20 minutes, or until light brown on top.

Avocado Tuna Melt Bites

Nutrition Info.
Calories: 135
Fats: 11.8g
Net carbs: 0.8g

Protein: 6.2g

Ingredients:
- Ten (10) oz. canned tuna, drained
- One quarter (1/4) cup mayonnaise
- One (1) medium avocado, cubed
- One quarter (1/4) cup parmesan cheese
- One third (1/3) cup almond flour
- Half (1/2) tsp. garlic powder
- One quarter (1/4) tsp. onion powder
- Salt and pepper to taste
- Half (1/2) cup coconut oil, from frying (~1/4 cup absorbed)

Instructions:
1. Drain a can of tuna and add it to a large container, where you will be able to mix everything together.
2. Add mayonnaise, parmesan cheese and spices to the tuna and mix well.
3. Slice an avocado in half, remove the pit and cube the inside
4. Add avocado to the tuna mixture and fold, trying to not mash the avocado into the

mixture.

5. Form the tuna mixture into balls and roll into almond flour, covering and set aside.
6. Heat coconut oil in a pan over medium heat. Once hot, add tuna balls and fry until crisp on all sides. Remove from the pan and serve.

Keto Mixed Green Spring Salad

Nutrition Info.
Calories: 478
Fats: 37.3g
Net carbs: 4.3g
Protein: 17.2g
Ingredients:
- Two (2) oz. mixed greens
- Three (3) tbsp. pine nuts, roasted
- Two (2) tbsp. 5 minute keto raspberry vinaigrette
- Two (2) tbsp. shaved parmesan
- Two (2) slices bacon
- Salt and pepper to taste

Instructions:
1. In a large frying pan, fry the bacon until very crisp.
2. Measure your greens and set in a container that can be shaken
3. Crumble bacon and then add the rest of the ingredients to the greens. Shake the container with a lid on to distribute the dressing and contents evenly.

Cheese Stuffed Bacon Wrapped Hot Dogs

Nutrition Info.
- Calories: 380
- Fats: 34.5g
- Net carbs: 0.3g
- Protein: 16.8g

Ingredients:
- Six (6) hot dogs
- Twelve (12) slices bacon
- Two (2) oz. cheddar cheese
- Half (1/2) tsp. onion powder

- Half (1/2) tsp. garlic powder
- Salt and pepper to taste

Instructions:
1. Pre-heat the oven to 400F. Make a cut, lengthwise, in all of the hot dogs to make room for the cheese.
2. Slice 2 oz. Cheddar cheese from a block into small, long rectangles and stuff into the hot dogs.
3. Continue tightly wrapping the second slice of bacon around the hot dog, slightly overlapping the first slice. It should resemble the traditional pigs in a blanket.
4. Poke toothpicks through each side of the bacon and hot dog, securing the bacon in place.
5. Set on a wire rack that is on top of a cookie sheet. Season with garlic powder, onion powder, salt, and pepper.
6. Bake for 35-40 minutes or until bacon is crispy. Additionally, broil the bacon on top.

Served with delicious creamed spinach.

Crisp Tofu and Bok Choy Salad

Nutrition Info.
- Calories: 442
- Fats: 35g
- Net carbs: 5.7g
- Protein:25g

Ingredients:
Oven Baked Tofu
- Fifteen (15) oz.eExtra firm Tofu
- One (1) tbsp. soy sauce
- One () tbsp. sesame oil
- One (1) tbsp. water
- Two (2) tsp. minced garlic
- One (1) tbsp. rice wine vinegar
- Juice half (1/2) lemon

Bok Choy Salad
- Nine (9) oz. bok choy
- One (1) stalk green onion
- Two (2) tbsp. cilantro, chopped
- Three (3) tbsp. coconut oil

- Two (2) tbsp. soy sauce
- One (1) tbsp. sambal olek
- One (1) tbsp. peanut butter
- Juice half (1/2) lime
- Seven (7) drops liquid stevia

Instructions:
1. Dry the tofu, known as pressing the tofu. Lay the tofu on a kitchen towel and put something heavy over the top (like a cast iron skillet). Keep an eye on the kitchen towel; it may be too full. Pressing will take between 4-6 hours.
2. Once the tofu is pressed, work on your marinade. In a small bowl, combine the soy sauce, sesame oil, water, garlic, viegar, and lemon.
3. Chop the tofu into squares and place these into a plastic bag with the marinade. Let this marinate for at least 30 minutes, but preferably overnight.
4. Pre-heat oven to 350F. Using parchment

paper, line a baking sheet. The tofu must be placed on this paper and put in the oven to bake for 30-35 minutes.

5. Mix all of the other ingredients (except lime juice and Bok Choy) in a bowl. Then add cilantro and spring onion.
6. Once the tofu is almost cooked, add lime juice into the salad dressing and mix.
7. Chop the Bok Choy into small slices, like cabbage. Remove the tofu from the oven and assemble your salad with tofu, Bok Choy, and sauce.

Ketogenic NasiLemak

Nutrition Info.
- Calories: 501.7
- Fats: 39.9g
- Net carbs: 6.9g
- Protein: 28.1g

Ingredients:
Fried Chicken:
- Two (2) boneless chicken thighs

- Half (1/2) tsp. curry powder
- One quarter (1/4) tsp. turmeric powder
- Half (1/2) tsp. lime juice
- One eight (1/8) tsp. salt
- Half (1/2) tsp. coconut oil

NasiLemak:
- Three (3) tbsp. coconut milk (from the can)
- Three (3) slices ginger
- Half (1/2) small shallot, sliced
- One quarter (1/4) tsp. salt (or to taste)
- Seven (7) oz. riced cauliflower
- Four (4) slices cucumber

Fried Egg:
- One (1) large egg
- Half (1/2) tbsp. unsalted butter

Instructions:
1. Prepare 7 oz. cauliflower rice (by ricing cauliflower and squeeze out water. To rice your cauliflower, pulse it in a food processor until it reaches your desired consistency. Set aside.

2. Marinade 2 boneless chicken thighs with ½ tsp. curry powder, ¼ tsp. turmeric powder, ½ tsp. lime juice and ½ tsp. salt. Set aside.
3. Fry the marinated chicken thighs until brown.
4. To prepare the rice, boil in a saucepan on medium heat: 3 tbsp. coconut milk, 3 slices ginger, ½ small shallot, and ¼ tsp. salt (or to taste). It should take about a minute or less.
5. Add the riced cauliflower and mix well. Once bubbling.
6. Serve with 2 slices cucumber and fried egg, with 1 tbsp. sambal and 1 chicken thigh.

Taco meat.

Nutrition Info:

Calories 259

Calories from Fat 90

Fat 10g15%

Saturated Fat 5g31%

Cholesterol 70mg23%

Sodium 321mg14%

Potassium 734mg21%

Carbohydrates 14g5%

Fiber 4g17%

Sugar 2g2%

Protein 28g56%.

Ingredients:

- 1 tbsp. vegetable oil
- 1 lbs. lean ground beef (5% fat)
- 1 onion, chopped
- 3 cloves garlic, pressed
- 2 tbsp. cumin
- 2 tsp dried coriander
- 1 tsp chili powder
- 1 tsp oregano
- 2 tbsp. tomato paste
- 125ml/1/2cup water
- salt to taste

- 170g/1cup canned black beans, blended in a food processor or blender.

Directions:

1. Heat the oil in a large pan and salute chopped onions over low heat for 5-7 minutes, then add the pressed garlic and cook for 30 seconds longer. Add the ground beef and brown until no longer pink. (Drain the fat if not using lean beef.)
2. To the beef add cumin, dried coriander, chili powder, oregano, tomato paste and water with a pinch of salt, turn the heat up and bring to a boil, then lower the heat, cover with a lid and let it simmer for 15 minutes.
3. Process the black bean with the liquid in a blender or food processor until smooth. Add to the beef and let it simmer uncovered for 10 minutes longer until most of the liquid has been absorbed by the beef. Taste the taco meat and add more salt if necessary.

Recipes substitutions

Any beans will work in place of black beans. I have successfully used red kidney beans, butter beans and chickpeas.

You can also use refried beans.

I prefer using extra lean beef but feel free to use 10% fat beef or higher if desired.

Eggplant Burgers

Nutrition Info.
- Calories: 426
- Fats: 23g
- Net carbs: 11g
- Protein: 28g

Ingredients:
- Half (1/2) cup/ 155 ground beef
- One (1) clove garlic finely chopped
- One quarter (1/4) small onion finely chopped
- One (1) pinch of sage powder
- One (1) pinch of salt
- Olive oil for sautéing beef

- One (1) tbsp./14 gr parmesan cheese
- One quarter (1/4) bunch/50 gr spinach

Egg Mixture
- One (1) small egg, beaten
- One (1) pinch of sage powder
- One (1) teaspoon of oregano
- One (1) pinch of cayenne powder optional

Eggplant mixture
- One (1) medium eggplant
- One (1) pinch onion powder
- On (1) pinch garlic powder
- One (1) pinch of salt

Instructions:
1. Slice eggplant in two parts and open in half. Season with salt and let it sit for 15 to 30 minutes. Wash before roasting
2. In a hot skillet with olive oil, sauté onions, and garlic. Add ground beef and slightly season with salt, ground pepper and sage. Brown meat without burning. Drain and transfer meat to platter.
3. Transfer eggplant to a non-stick baking

tray. Season ground black pepper. Drizzle some olive oil before roasting.

4. In a pre-heated 350 degrees F./180 degrees C oven, roast eggplant slices for 12 to 15 minutes until soft. Allow to cool, then discard skin. Cut in small pieces or slivers. Season well with onion powder and garlic powder. Mix well

5. In a bowl, beat the egg. Season with sage, oregano, and salt. Opt to add cayenne for a little heat

6. Combine eggplant mixture to cooked ground beef. Add egg mixture. Mix well

7. In the same skillet, heat oil and drop egg rings. Pour two to three tablespoons of eggplant and beef mixture to fill the egg rings and flatten with the back of a spoon. Cover skillet. Allow for eggplant burger patties to form for about two minutes.

8. Slowly remove eggrings and flip the patties, the way you flip an ordinary burger or pancake. Cook for 1 to 2

minutes. Allow for excess oil to drip and transfer to a serving platter. Do this to the remaining patties. Cover with parmesan shredded cheese

Keto Lasagnas

Nutrition Info.
- Calories: 329
- Fats: 25g
- Net carbs: 4.25g
- Protein: 22g

Ingredients:
- One quarter (1/4) cup/ 57 gr ricotta cheese
- One (1) tbsp./ 14 gr parmesan cheese
- One (1) tbsp. mozzarella cheese, shredded
- One (1) small egg
- Half (1/2) clove of garlic
- One quarter (1/4) cup lean ground beef, cooked
- One (1) tablespoon/ 14 gr tomato sauce

- One (1) pinch of pink salt
- One (1) teaspoon of coconut oil or ghee
- One quarter (1/4) large zucchini

Instructions:
1. Add coconut oil to a medium high pan and cook the ground beef. Add the tomato sauce to the ground beef and combine
2. Using a mandolin slicer, slice the zucchini into as many thin slices as possible
3. Add the ricotta, parmesan, garlic cloves, salt, pepper, and egg to a processor and blend until fully combined
4. In an oven one portion skillet or casserole dish first make a layer of the ground beef
5. Make two layers of the zucchini criss crossing
6. Add a generous layer of the ricotta mixture
7. Sprinkle on some of the shredded mozzarella.
8. Repeat this a second time. Last layer

should be the mozzarella cheese.
9. Bake in a 350 degrees F oven for 30 minutes or until cheese is browned.

Fresh Cheese & Grilled Zucchini

Nutrition Info.
- Calories: 818
- Fats: 70g
- Total carbs: 7.1
- Net carbs: 6.2
- Protein: 45.2g

Ingredients:
- Half (1/2) cup fresh Robiola cheese
- Half (1/2) cup mozzarella cheese
- Half (1/2) cup fresh zucchini, thinly sliced
- One (1) tablespoon of olive oil
- One (1) tsp. of fresh garlic, chopped
- One (1) tsp. of fresh parsley, chopped
- One (1) pinch of salt
- One (1) pinch of white pepper

Instructions:

1. Grill the finely chopped zucchini on a grill, sprinkling with half of the garlic. Once ready season with salt and pepper and dash of raw oil
2. Spread the Robiola at the center of a plate and cover up with thin slices of mozzarella and sprinkle with the remaining garlic
3. Put plate in the microwave for 5 seconds on "grill" mode, until the mozzarella has started to melt
4. Surround the cheese by the zucchini and season to serve.

Sautéed Shrimp

Ingredients:
- Half (1/2) pound shrimp, peeled and deveined
- One (1) tablespoon freshly squeezed lemon juice
- One (1) tablespoon chopped parsley
- One (1) teaspoon of olive oil
- Half (1/2) teaspoon herb seasoning

- Salt and pepper to taste

Instruction:
- Place skillet over medium heat and add oil.
- Stir in shrimp and sauté for one minute.
- Sprinkle with salt, herb seasoning and pepper.
- Drizzle with lemon juice and keep stirring.
- Cook for four minutes
- Sprinkle chopped parsley before transferring to a serving dish.

Beef with Broccoli

Ingredients:
- One quarter (1/4) pound round steak, cut into thick strips
- One quarter (1/4) onion, sliced into wedges
- One (1) cup broccoli florets
- One eight (1/8) cup water
- One (1) tbsp. cornstarch
- One (1) tbsp. of soy sauce

- One (1) tbsp. vegetable oil
- One (1) tbsp. water, divided
- One quarter(1/4) teaspoon ground ginger
- One eight (1/8) teaspoon garlic powder

Instructions:
1. Mix garlic powder, cornstarch and water in a bowl. Add the steak strips. Mix well.
2. Place a skillet over medium heat and pour half the oil portion.
3. Add coated beefs strips and stir fry until tender.
4. Transfer the beef strips onto a plate.
5. Then, pour other half portion of oil into the skillet and cook the onion and broccoli.
6. Cook for 4 minutes. Add the beef strips back into the skillet and add brown sugar, ginger, cornstarch, soy sauce and water.
7. Stir fry for another 2 minutes. Serve immediately.

Green Beans with Bacon.

Nutritional Info:

258 calories

8g fat

Carbs 36g

Protein 129

Ingredients:
- 2 pounds of green beans (fresh)
- 8 strips bacon (diced)
- 3 tablespoons butter
- Black pepper (to taste)
- Salt (to taste)

Directions:
1. Gather the ingredients.
2. Wash the green beans in a colander under cold running water.
3. Top and tail them (slice off the stem ends and tail ends) and then cut them into 1- to 1 1/2-inch pieces. Set aside.

4. Heat a large skillet or sauté pan over medium heat; add the diced bacon. Fry the bacon until crispy.
5. Remove the bacon to paper towels to drain.
6. Leave 2 to 3 tablespoons (or more) of the bacon drippings in skillet and save the remaining drippings for another recipe. Set the skillet aside.
7. Bring a pot of salted water to boil over high heat and then add the beans. Boil for about 8 to 12 minutes, or until the desired doneness is reached.
8. Drain the green beans well and then add them to the skillet along with cooked bacon and butter. Toss well and heat until the green beans are thoroughly coated and hot.
9. Sprinkle the green beans with freshly ground black pepper and salt, to taste.
10. Serve with your choice, and enjoy!

Yummy Eggplant Burgers

Nutrition Info.
Calories: 426 (2 burgers per serving)
Fat: 23g
Total carbs: 22g
Net carbs: 11g
Protein: 28g

Ingredients:
- Half (½) cup ground beef
- One (1) clove garlic finely chopped
- One quarter (1/4) small onion finely chopped
- One (1) pinch of sage powder
- One (1) pinch of salt
- Olive oil for sautéing beef
- One (1) tbsp. parmesan cheese
- One quarter (1/4) bunch spinach

Egg Mixture:
- One (1) small egg, beaten
- One (1) pinch of sage powder
- One (1) teaspoon of oregano
- One (1) pinch of cayenne powder

(optional)

Eggplant Mixture:
- One (1) medium eggplant
- One (1) pinch onion powder
- One (1) pinch garlic powder
- One (1) pinch of salt

Instructions:
1. Slice eggplant in two parts and open in half. Use salt to season and let it sit for fifteen-thirty minutes. Wash before roasting.
2. Use a hot skillet with olive oil to sauté the onions and garlic. Add ground beef and use salt, ground pepper, and sage to lightly season.
3. Brown meat without burning. Drain and transfer meat to a platter
4. Move eggplant to a non-stick baking tray. Season ground black pepper. Drizzle some olive oil before roasting.
5. Roast eggplant slices for twelve-fifteen minutes until soft in a pre-heated 350

degrees F/180 degrees C oven.

6. Let it cool off, then discard skin. Cut in small pieces or slivers. Use onion powder and garlic powder to season well.
7. Beat the egg in a bowl. Season with sage, oregano, and salt. Opt to add cayenne for a little heat.
8. Add up eggplant mixture to cooked ground beef. Add egg mixture. Mix thoroughly.
9. In the same skillet, heat oil and drop egg rings. Pour two-three tablespoons of eggplant and beef mixture to fill the egg rings and flatten with the back of a spoon. Cover skillet. Allow for eggplant burger patties to form for about two minutes.
10. Gently remove egg rings and flip the patties, the same way you flip an ordinary burger or pancake. Cook for one-two minutes. Allow excess oil to drip and transfer to a serving platter.
11. Do this with the balance patties. Cover with parmesan shredded cheese.

Greek Chicken Salad

Ingredients:
- Half (½) cooked chicken breast, cut into bite-size pieces
- One quarter (1/4) cup crumbled feta cheese
- Half (½) medium cucumber, peeled, seeded, and chopped
- One quarter (1/4) cup pitted green olives
- One quarter (1/4) cup cherry tomatoes, halved
- Three (3) tbsp. homemade mayonnaise
- Two (2) tbsp. minced onion

Directions:
1. In a bowl, combine the chicken, feta, cucumber, olives, and tomatoes.
2. Add the mayonnaise and minced. Mix very well.

Cranberry Walnut Salad

Nutrition Info:
Calories: 282
Fat: 17.1g
Total carbs: 6.6g
Net carbs: 2.1g
Protein: 26.8g

Ingredients:
- Half (½)/ 1oo g cooked chicken breast
- Half (½) stalk celery chopped
- One (1) tbsp. unsweetened dried cranberries
- One (1) tbsp. walnuts chopped
- Half (½) small avocado, ripe
- One (1) dash of lemon juice
- One (1) pinch of salt

Instructions:
1. Dice up cooked chicken. In a large bowl mix together chicken, celery, cranberries, and walnuts.
2. Mash avocados with lemon juice and pepper in a separate small bowl.
3. Stir avocado mixture into chicken mix.

Season with salt to taste.

Watermelon, Mint & Feta Salad

Ingredients:
- One (1) cup watermelon, cut into bite-size cubes
- One (1) medium cucumber, peeled, seeded and chopped
- Four (4) oz. feta cheese, crumbled
- One third (1/3) cup walnuts
- One (1) handful fresh mint leaves, chopped

Directions:
1. Gently combine all the ingredients together. Mix very well.
2. Chill for two hours before serving.

Pork Tenderloin

Nutrition Info.
Calories: 223
Fat: 5.8g
Total carbs: 8.3g

Net carbs: 5.3g
Protein: 20.3g

Ingredients:
- One (1) dash olive oil
- One (1) clove garlic minced
- Two (2) slices pork tenderloin
- One (1) dash balsamic vinegar
- One (1) tsp. Worcestershire sauce
- One (1) tsp. coconut aminos
- One (1) pinch of salt
- One (1) pinch of red pepper flakes
- Half (½) cup broccoli, steamed

Instructions:
1. Drizzle your olive oil onto the bottom of crock pot. Sprinkle in garlic, and then roll pork tenderloin into it.
2. Combine the remaining ingredients in a small bowl and pour over pork.
3. Cover and cook on high for three-four hours or low four-six hours
4. Steam the broccoli until bright green but

tender

5. Remove meat to serving the dish and pour about half cup of juice over the meat. Reserve the rest of the juice to pour over individual servings.

Beef And Broccoli.

Nutrition Info:

Calories; 331

Fat; 21.1g

Cholesterol; 52 mg

Sodium; 419 mg

Carbohydrates; 13.3 g

Protein; 21.7 g

Ingredients:

- ⅓ cup oyster sauce
- 2 teaspoons Asian (toasted) sesame oil
- ⅓ cup sherry
- 1 teaspoon soy sauce
- 1 teaspoon white sugar
- 1 teaspoon cornstarch

- ¾ pound beef round steak, cut into 1/8-inch thick strips
- 3 tablespoons vegetable oil, plus more if needed
- 1 thin slice of fresh ginger root
- 1 clove garlic, peeled and smashed
- 1 pound broccoli, cut into florets

Directions:

1. Whisk together the oyster sauce, sesame oil, sherry, soy sauce, sugar, and cornstarch in a bowl, and stir until the sugar has dissolved.
2. Place the steak pieces into a shallow bowl, pour the oyster sauce mixture over the meat, stir to coat well, and marinate for at least 30 minutes in the refrigerator.
3. Heat vegetable oil in a wok or large skillet over medium-high heat, and stir in the ginger and garlic. Let them sizzle in the hot oil for about 1 minute to flavor the oil, then remove and discard. Stir in the broccoli, and toss and stir in hot oil until

bright green and almost tender, 5 to 7 minutes. Remove the broccoli from the wok, and set aside.

4. Pour a little more oil into the wok, if needed, and stir and toss the beef with the marinade until the sauce forms a glaze on the beef, and the meat is no longer pink, about 5 minutes. Return the cooked broccoli to the wok, and stir until the meat and broccoli are heated through, about 3 minutes.

Snacks And Sides for After 50: Asparagus Fries.

Nutrition Info:

Calories: 177

Total Fat: 5 g

Saturated Fat: 2 g

Fat: 0 g

Cholesterol: 53 mg

Sodium: 269 mg

Carbohydrates: 24 g

Dietary Fiber: 2 g

Sugars: 2 g

Protein: 10 g.

Ingredients:

- 20 pieces asparagus spears, hard ends taken away
- 1/2 cup flour
- 1 egg
- 1/2 cup whole grain breadcrumbs
- 1/3 cup Parmesan cheese, grated.

Directions:

1. Preheat the oven to 400 degrees F.
2. Dip the asparagus in the flour then shake off the excess. Dip it next to the egg then the breadcrumbs. Shake off the excess.
3. Place them on a baking tray lined with baking paper then bake them for 10 minutes.
4. Take them out of the oven then sprinkle the Parmesan cheese on top.
5. Bake for another 10 minutes or until they are golden brown.

Kale chips.

Nutrition Info:

Calories; 58

Fat; 2.8g

Carbohydrates; 7.6g

Protein; 2.5g

Cholesterol; 0 mg

Sodium. 185 mg

Ingredients:
- 1 bunch kale
- 1 tablespoon olive oil
- 1 teaspoon seasoned salt

Directions:
1. Preheat an oven to 350 degrees F (175 degrees C). Line a non-insulated cookie sheet with parchment paper.
2. With a knife or kitchen shears carefully remove the leaves from the thick stems and tear into bite size pieces. Wash and thoroughly dry kale with a salad spinner.

Drizzle kale with olive oil and sprinkle with seasoning salt.

3. Bake until the edges brown but are not burnt, 10 to 15 minutes

Chocó Roasted Almonds

Nutrition Info.
Calories: 196
Fat: 15.8g
Total carbs: 7.6g
Net carbs: 2.8g
Protein: 6.8g

Ingredients:
- Thirty (30) grams raw almonds
- One (1) tsp. unsweetened dark cocoa powder
- One (1) tsp. Stevia powder
- One (1) pinch of Himalayan salt

Directions:
1. Spread the almonds onto a baking sheet and roast at 300 degrees for twenty minutes

2. In a bowl, put the roasted almonds and add the cocoa powder and stevia powder. Mix well.
3. Place the coated almond out in an even layer back on the baking sheet to cool. Store in a sealable container for up to six months.

Cheese Crackers

Nutrition Info
Calories: 512
Fat: 40.4g
Total carbs: 1.4g
Net carbs: 1.4g
Protein: 34.4g

Ingredients:
- Half (½) cup Swiss cheese
- One (1) tsp. oregano

Instructions:
1. Preheat your oven to 350 degrees F. and use a baking paper to cover the baking tray

2. Put some slice of the hard cheese on the baking tray.
3. Bake for ten-twelve minutes in the oven until the cheese has a brown color.
4. Take a paper towel and use it to absorb the excess oil and let it cool.

Peanut Butter Smoothie

Nutrition Info.
Calories: 287
Fat: 19.33g
Total carbs: 10.92g
Net carbs: 4.34g
Protein: 23.5g

Ingredients:
- One third (1/3) cup of silk original unsweetened almond milk
- One (1) cup of rice
- One (1) tbsp. unsweetened natural peanut butter
- One (1) tbsp. Chocó-flavored whey protein powder

- One (1) tbsp. heavy whipping cream
- One (1) pinch of vanilla extract
- One (1) tsp. Stevia powder (optional)

Instructions:

1. Pour almond milk into the blender and add rice, whey powder, peanut butter, vanilla extract, cream, and stevia powder. Blend until smooth and pour into glass.

Salami Cheese Roll-ups

Ingredients:
- Four (4) slices salami
- Four (4) slices mild cheddar cheese (totaling 1 oz.)

Directions:

1. Lay each slice of salami on a slice of cheese. Roll up and enjoy!

Blue Cheese & Strawberries

Ingredients:

- Two (2) oz. blue cheese
- Half (½) cup strawberries

Directions:
1. Divide the strawberries lengthwise into thick slices.
2. Thinly slice the blue cheese and eat each piece with a slice of strawberry.

Keto Chocolate Pudding

Nutrition Info.
Calories: 402
Fat: 20.3g
Total carbs: 12.09g
Net carbs: 4.47g
Protein: 3.25g

Ingredients:
- Two (2) cups coconut milk
- Two (2) tbsp. erythritol
- Two (2) tbsp. bitter cola powder
- Two (2) tsp. glucomannan powder

Instructions:

1. Add milk with cocoa and sweetener. Join glucomannan slowly to avoid lumps.
2. Put in microwave wave for one and half minutes, avoiding high-temperature mode boiling.
3. Place in the fridge for few hours, until it's cold.
4. Garnish with 99% dark chocolate chips. Enjoy!

Blueberry Mug Cake

Nutrition Info.
Calories: 219
Fat: 19.5g
Total carbs: 6.2g
Net carbs: 3.7g
Protein: 5.4g

Ingredients:
- Two (2) tbsp. almond flour
- One (1) tbsp. coconut flour
- One quarter (1/4) tsp. baking powder
- One (1) dash salt

- One (1) tbsp. fresh or frozen blueberries
- One (1) tbsp. coconut oil melted
- One (1) tbsp. heavy cream
- One (1) small egg
- One (1) tsp. natural stevia
- One (1) pinch vanilla extract
- One (1) pinch lemon extract

Directions:
1. In a small bowl, combine almond flour, coconut flour, baking powder, and salt. Mix well. Stir in blueberries.
2. In a small microwave bowl, melt coconut oil. Beat in heavy cream, egg, sweetener, and extracts into melted coconut.
3. Use a fork to beat dry ingredients into the liquid ingredients until well combined.
4. Divide batter between two lightly buttered ramekins. Microwave on high from 1 ½-2 minutes or until cake is no longer wet.

Guacamole

Nutrition Info:

Calories; 45

Fat; 3.7g

Carbohydrates; 3.4g

Protein; 0.7g

Cholesterol 0 mg

Sodium. 2mg

Ingredients:

- 2 avocados
- 1 small onion, finely chopped
- 1 clove garlic, minced
- 1 ripe tomato, chopped
- 1 lime, juiced salt and pepper to taste.

Directions:

1. Peel and mash avocados in a medium serving bowl.
2. Stir in onion, garlic, tomato, lime juice, salt and pepper.

3. Season with remaining lime juice and salt and pepper to taste. Chill for half an hour to blend flavors.

Zucchini Noodles

Nutrition Info:

Calories; 157

Fat; 13.9

Carbohydrates; 7.9g

Protein; 2.9g

Cholesterol; 0 mg

Sodium.181 mg

Ingredients:

- 2 zucchini, peeled
- 1 tablespoon olive oil
- 1/4 cup water
- salt and ground black pepper to taste

Directions:

1. Cut lengthwise slices from zucchini using a vegetable peeler, stopping when the seeds are reached. Turn zucchini over and

continue 'peeling' until all the zucchini is in long strips; discard seeds. Slice the zucchini into thinner strips resembling spaghetti.
2. Heat olive oil in a skillet over medium heat; cook and stir zucchini in the hot oil for 1 minute. Add water and cook until zucchini is softened, 5 to 7 minutes. Season with salt and pepper

Cauliflower Soufflé.

Nutrition Info:

Calories 172

Fat 11g17%

Saturated Fat 5g31%

Cholesterol 149mg50%

Sodium 225mg10%

Potassium 501mg14%

Carbohydrates 8g3%

Fiber 2g8%

Sugar 3g3%

Protein 11g22%

Ingredients:

- 1 head fresh cauliflower chopped, cooked and mashed
- ¾ cup finely shredded mozzarella
- 3 eggs
- 2 tbsps. heavy cream
- 2 tbsps. fresh parsley chopped
- salt and black pepper

Directions:

1. Preheat the oven to 350F.
2. Add the mashed cauliflower to a bowl, then add the remaining ingredients. Stir well to combine.
3. Pour mixture into an oven-safe dish and bake for 30-35 minutes until puffed and golden brown.

Strawberry Avocado Mousse

Nutrition Info.
Calories: 355
Fat: 35.2g
Total carbs: 10g
Net carbs: 2g

Protein: 6.1g

Ingredients:
- Half (½) medium avocado
- One (1) tbsp. whey protein, strawberry flavor
- One (1) tbsp. cream
- One (1) pinch pure vanilla extract
- Two (2) tbsp. water
- Three (3) cubes of ice

Instructions:
1. Combine everything with a kitchen robot, adding cubes of ice.
2. Place in the refrigerator for an hour to thicken it.
3. If the mousse is too thick, you can use one tablespoon of unsweetened soy milk to mix it.

Egg Mayo

Nutrition Info.
Calories: 211

Fat: 17g
Total carbs: 0.76
Net carbs: 0.76
Protein: 13.05g

Ingredients:
- One (1) small boiled egg
- One (1) tbsp. mayonnaise
- Salt and pepper

Instructions:
1. Divide the egg in half and use the mayonnaise to garnish. Season to pleasure.

Green Smoothie

Ingredients:
- One (1) tbsp. MCT Oil
- One (1) tbsp. flax meal
- One (1) tbsp. chia seeds
- Half (½) a scoop vanilla whey protein
- One (1) cup frozen spinach
- One (1) tbsp. cocoa butter

- Cubes Ice
- Three (3) cups water

Instructions:
1. Add all ingredients in a blender and mix on high for about thirty seconds, or until spinach is mostly liquefied

Almond Butter Fudge

Ingredients:
- One (1) cup almond butter (unsweetened)
- One (1) cup coconut oil
- One quarter (1/4) cup coconut milk
- One (1) tsp. vanilla extract
- Stevia to taste

Directions:
1. Dissolve the almond butter and coconut oil so that they can become softened.
2. Add all the ingredients and blend very well.
3. Pour the blended mixture into a pan and place in the fridge for two-three hours for

it to be ready.

4. Before serving, cut into chunks.

Chocolate Hazelnut Smoothie

Ingredients:
- One (1) tbsp. cocoa powder
- One quarter (1/4) cup hazelnuts
- One third (1/3) cup heavy cream
- Two (2) tbsp. low-carb chocolate protein powder
- One (1) tbsp. MCT oil
- Water

Directions:
1. Combine all ingredients and blend until smooth.

Aztec Chocolate Smoothie

Ingredients:
- Two (2) tbsp. cocoa powder
- One (1) avocado
- Two (2) tbsp. low-carb chocolate protein

powder
- Half (½) tsp. cinnamon
- Four (4) tsp. MCT oil
- Pinch chili powder
- Water

Directions:
Add all ingredients and blend until smooth.

Blackberry Coconut Fat Bombs

Nutrition Info
Calories: 170
Fat: 18.7g
Total carbs: 3g
Net carbs: 0.7g
Protein: 1.1g

Ingredients:
- One (1) tbsp. coconut butter
- One (1) tbsp. coconut oil
- One (1) tbsp. fresh or frozen blackberries (you can also use raspberries or strawberries)
- One (1) pinch vanilla extract

- One (1) pinch natural stevia
- One (1) dash lemon juice

Instructions:
1. In a pot, put coconut butter, coconut oil and blackberries (if frozen) and heat over medium heat until well combined.
2. Add coconut oil mix and the balance ingredients in a food processor or blender. Process until well smooth. If you took the option of fresh berries, there is no point cooking them with coconut oil and butter.
3. Place into a small pan lined with parchment paper.
4. Put in the fridge for one hour or until the mix has hardened.

Strawberry Protein Smoothie

Nutrition Info.
Calories: 374
Fat: 31.37g
Total carbs: 8.54
Net carbs: 1.96

Protein: 20.81

Ingredients:
- One (1) tbsp. lactose-free mascarpone cheese
- One quarter (1/3) cup of Silk Original Unsweetened Almond milk
- One (1) cup rice
- One (1) tbsp. strawberry-flavored whey protein powder
- One (1) tbsp. heavy whipping cream
- One (1) tbsp. cocoa butter
- One (1) pinch of vanilla extract
- One (1) tsp. stevia powder (optional)

Instructions:
1. Pour the almond milk into a blender and add ice, whey powder, mascarpone, cream, vanilla extract, and stevia powder.
2. Blend until smooth and pour into glasses.

Almond Butter Balls

Ingredients:
- Two (2) tbsp. almond butter
- One (1) tbsp. vanilla almond whey protein or vanilla flavor (1 scoop)
- Two (2) tbsp. unsweetened flaked coconut
- One (1) tsp. sugar-free chocolate chips
- One (1) pinch natural stevia

Instructions:
1. In a medium bowl, combined all ingredients until well combined.
2. Scoop and form into balls about a tablespoon in size.
3. Cover and store in the fridge.

Berry Protein Smoothie

Nutrition Info.
Calories: 406
Fat: 30.5g
Total carbs: 10.05g
Net carbs: 7.5g
Protein: 21g

Ingredients:

- One (1) cup unsweetened almond milk
- One (1) cup rice
- One (1) tbsp. cocoa butter
- One (1) tbsp. coconut oil
- Two (2) tbsp. strawberry whey protein powder
- One third (1/3) cup blackberries
- One (1) tsp. xanthan gum
- One (1) tbsp. stevia powder
- One (1) tsp. pure vanilla extract

Instructions:
1. Empty the almond milk into a blender and add ice, then follow by other ingredients.
2. Blend until smooth and pour into glasses. Enjoy!

Cheddar Muffin

Nutrition Info.
Calories: 169.42
Fat: 10.62g
Total carbs: 5.14g
Net carbs: 2.14g

Protein: 10.5g

Ingredients:
- One (1) large egg
- Two (2) tbsp. coconut flour
- One (1) pinch baking soda
- One (1) pinch salt
- One (1) pinch of sweet paprika
- One (1) pinch of dried parsley
- One (1) tbsp. shredded cheddar

Instructions:
1. Use coconut oil to grease a dish or butter.
2. Use a fork to mix all ingredients together in a bowl and ensure it is smooth (saving a little bit of cheddar for topping).
3. Use the leftover shredded cheddar to top with it.
4. Put the dough in the greased dish and cook in the microwave on "high" for one minute. You can also use the oven to bake it at 180 degrees for fourteen minutes.

Keto Jelly

Nutrition Info.
Calories: 68
Fat: 6.8g
Total carbs: 1.6g
Net carbs: 1.6g
Protein: 0.8g

Ingredients:
- One quarter (1/4) cup coconut milk
- Half (½) tsp. agar agar (gelatine can be use also)
- Cherry aroma or bandy aroma
- One (1) tsp. stevia sweetener

Instructions:
1. Use a low flame to heat up the coconut milk with the aroma and sweetener.
2. Put in the agar agar and boil for three-four minutes.
3. Using a rectangular mold, pour in the mixture and allow it to cool until it becomes hard. Then cut in pieces (about

four slices).

Dinner Recipes for After 50:

Whole Chicken

Nutrition Info:

Calories; 423

Total fat; 32.1 g

Cholesterol; 97 mg

Sodium. 662 mg

Carbohydrates; 1.2 g

Protein.39.9 g

Ingredients:

- 1 (3 pound) whole chicken, giblets removed
- salt and black pepper to taste
- 1 tablespoon onion powder, or to taste
- ½ cup margarine, divided
- 1 stalk celery, leaves removed

Directions:

1. Preheat oven to 350 degrees F (175 degrees C).

2. Place chicken in a roasting pan, and season generously inside and out with salt and pepper. Sprinkle inside and out with onion powder. Place 3 tablespoons margarine in the chicken cavity. Arrange dollops of the remaining margarine around the chicken's exterior. Cut celery into 3 or 4 pieces, and place in the chicken cavity.
3. Bake uncovered 1 hour and 15 minutes in the preheated oven, to a minimum internal temperature of 180 degrees F (82 degrees C).
4. Remove from heat, and baste with melted margarine and drippings.
5. Cover with aluminum foil, and allow to rest for about 30 minutes before serving.

Lamb Shanks:

Nutrition Info:
Calories; 481
Fat; 21.8g
Carbohydrates; 17.6 g

Protein; 30.3 g

Cholesterol; 93 mg

Sodium; 759 mg

Ingredients:

- 6 lamb shanks salt and pepper to taste
- 2 tablespoons olive oil
- 2 onions, chopped
- 3 large carrots, cut into 1/4 inch rounds
- 10 cloves garlic, minced
- 1 (750 milliliter) bottle red wine
- 1 (28 ounce) can whole peeled tomatoes with juice
- 1 (10.5 ounce) can condensed chicken broth
- 1 (10.5 ounce) can beef broth
- 5 teaspoons chopped fresh rosemary
- 2 teaspoons chopped fresh thyme.

Directions:

1. Sprinkle shanks with salt and pepper. Heat oil in heavy large pot or Dutch oven over medium-high heat. Working in batches,

cook shanks until brown on all sides, about 8 minutes. Transfer shanks to plate.
2. Add onions, carrots and garlic to pot and salute until golden brown, about 10 minutes. Stir in wine, tomatoes, chicken broth and beef broth.
3. Season with rosemary and thyme. Return shanks to pot, pressing down to submerge. Bring to a boil, then reduce heat to medium-low. Cover, and simmer until meat is tender, about 2 hours.
4. Remove cover from pot. Simmer about 20 minutes longer. Transfer shanks to platter, place in a warm oven.
5. Boil juices in pot until thickened, about 15 minutes. Spoon over shanks.

Mushroom Stake

Ingredients:
- Half (½) cup beef stake
- One (1) cup boiled mushrooms
- One (1) tbsp. cream

- One (1) pinch of salt
- One (1) pinch of pepper

Instructions:
1. Preheat the oven to 250 degrees F.
2. Put salt and pepper on both sides of the steak. Heat a cast iron frying pan.
3. Use two minutes to cook the steaks on both sides, and then transfer to oven for finishing.
4. Cook in the oven until the internal temperature reaches the desired level.
5. Put the steak aside to rest once it is ready. Add a little port wine to the pan to blend and scrape some of the leftover meat residues
6. Add the mushrooms and some cream to the pan. Once the sauce is thickened, pour over the steak and serve.

(Calories: 366, fat: 25g, total carbs: 8g, net carbs: 5g, protein: 30.1g)

Keto Avocado Sushi

Ingredients:
- Half (½) nori wrapper
- Half (½) cup chopped cauliflower
- Half (½) cup cream cheese
- Half (½) small cucumber
- One quarter (1/4) medium avocado
- One (1) tsp. coconut oil
- Soy sauce (for dipping)

Instructions:
1. Cut up about the cauliflower into florets and pulse in processor until consistency of rice
2. Use a medium-high skillet to heat coconut oil, and add cauliflower rice.
3. Use five-seven minutes to cook until rice is slightly browned and fully cooked through. Put in a bowl.
4. Slice avocado, cream cheese and cucumber into thin slices and put aside with cauliflower.

(Calories: 230.75, fat: 22.15g, total carbs: 8.65g, net carbs: 4.23g, Protein: 4.45g

Romaine Saltimbocca Chicken

Ingredients:
- One quarter (1/4) chicken breasts
- One (1) slice prosciutto
- Two (2) tbsp. asiago cheese
- One (1) tbsp. frozen spinach
- One (1) tbsp. coconut oil
- One (1) tbsp. olive oil (for finishing)
- One (1) pinch of salt

Instructions:
1. Use a mallet to flatten out the chicken piece. Take the slice of prosciutto and place it on the piece of chicken.
2. Divide the spinach and asiago cheese evenly onto the piece of chicken.
3. Roll up the chicken and put a toothpick through the piece to hold it firmly during cooking.

4. Heat a pan over medium heat and add two tablespoons of coconut oil. Add the chicken when the oil is up to temperature.
5. Cook for about thirty minutes. They might take a while to cook due to their size, but ensure they are cook through.
6. Use the olive oil to drizzle over the top when serving.

(Calories: 431.7, fat: 28g, total carbs: 1.8g, net carbs: 1.3g, protein: 45.7g

Stake & ghee Broccoli

Ingredients:
- One (1) ribeye steak
- One (1) pinch of salt
- Paprika to taste
- Onion powder to taste
- Garlic powder to taste
- One (1) tbsp. avocado oil
- Half (½) cup broccoli
- Two (2) tbsp. ghee

Instructions:
1. Use foil to cover the baking tray and top off with a metal rack.
2. Boil broccoli. Sprinkle seasonings on the steak to taste. Then place meat on a rack
3. Bake steak in 275 degrees F preheated oven until meat reaches a temperature of 125 degrees F in the center (about forty-fifty minutes).
4. Bring out the steak from the oven, use foil to cover and let it sit five-ten minutes while heating oiled cast iron pan on high.
5. Sear the steak for a minute on each side. Heat up broccoli on a skillet melting ghee on top.

(Calories: 441, fat: 33g, total carbs: 7g, net carbs: 4g, protein: 29g)

Keto Hot Salami Pizza

Ingredients:
- One quarter (1/4) cup mozzarella cheese, shredded

- One (1) tbsp. cream cheese
- One (1) small egg
- One (1) tbsp. almond flour

For the topping:
- One (1) tbsp. tomato sauce (sugarless)
- Three (3) thin slices of hot salami (4" dia x 1/8" thick)
- One (1) pinch of oregano
- One (1) pinch of salt

Instructions:
1. Preheat oven to 425 degrees.
2. In a bowl, add the mozzarella cheese and cream cheese and microwave for thirty seconds.
3. Bring it out of microwave and mix. Microwave for thirty seconds more and mix again.
4. Add your almond flour and egg to the melted mixture. Combine all the ingredients and mix with a fork until they are well combined and begin to cool.
5. Knead by hand and form into a pizza crust

on a nonstick pan.

6. Bake for 12-14 minutes at 425 degrees F. bring it out from the oven, add desired toppings and bake for an extra five-seven minute.

(calories: 721, fat: 56.89g, total carbs: 10g, net carbs: 7g, protein: 42.6g)

Superfood Soup with Air Cured Beef

Ingredients:
- Half (½) small onion
- Half (½) bunch of spinach
- Half (½) cup coconut milk
- Half (½) cup bresaola air cured beef
- One (1) small celery stalk
- One (1) clove garlic
- One (1) tbsp. coconut oil
- One (1) pinch of bay leaf

Instructions:
1. Finely peel and dice onion and garlic and put in a pot with clarified butter and

coconut oil.
2. Use a medium to high heat to cook until a bit golden.
3. Dice your vegetables and put it in the pot with the browned onion. Add crumbled laurel leaf.
4. Cook it for approximately five minutes and mix constantly.
5. Then, add your spinach and cook until dried for approximately two-three minutes.
6. Pour a liter of vegetable broth and bring to a boil. Stir in the coconut milk and season with salt and pepper.
7. Bring it out from the fire and make cream with a blender.

Ham & Cheese Pizza with Asparagus

Ingredients:
- One (1) slice uncured smoked ham
- One (1) tbsp. tomato sauce or pizza sauce
- One (1) slice mozzarella
- One (1) tsp. ghee

- Half (½) cup asparagus

Instructions:
1. On a rimmed baking sheet, lay out the ham slices.
2. Use a tablespoon of sauce to spread on each sauce.
3. Use a slice of cheese to top each ham slice.
4. Put under broiler (or in 400 degrees F oven) until cheese is browned.

Stake & Marinated Zucchini

Ingredients:
- Half (½) cup ribeye steak
- One (1) pinch of salt
- One (1) pinch of sweet paprika
- One (1) pinch of onion powder
- One pinch (1) pinch of garlic powder
- One (1) tbsp. avocado oil
- Half (½) cup zucchini
- One (1) pinch of parsley

Instructions:
1. Use foil to cover baking tray and top off with a metal rack.
2. Add seasonings on steak to taste. Place meat on rack.
3. Bake steak in 275 degrees F. preheated oven until meat reaches a temperature of 125 degrees F. in the center (approximately 40-50 minutes).
4. Bring out the steak from the oven, use foil to cover it and let it sit five-ten minutes while heating oiled cast iron pan on high.
5. Sear the steak for a minute on each side.

(Calories: 574, fat: 44.03g, total carbs: 3.8g, net carbs: 2.8g, protein: 42.2g)

Baked Trout Fillets with Sour Cream & Broccoli

Ingredients:
- One (1) trout fillet
- One (1) tbsp. sour cream
- One (1) dash lemon juice
- One (1) dash garlic powder

- One (1) pinch of salt
- One (1) pinch of paprika
- Half (½) cup broccoli

Instructions:
1. Boil the broccoli. In a greased shallow baking dish, place cured fish.
2. Add the sour cream, lemon juice, onion and salt in a small bowl, spread over fish. Sprinkle with paprika.
3. Bake, uncovered, at 350 degrees F. for 20-25 minutes or until fish flakes easily with a fork.

(Calories: 260, fat: 17g, total carbs: 9g, net carbs: 6g, protein: 20g)

Pizza Chicken Skillet

Ingredients:
- One (1) tsp. avocado oil or olive oil
- Half (½) cup skinless/boneless chicken piece
- One (1) pinch of salt
- Half (½) clove garlic minced

- One quarter (1/4) cup low carb pizza or marinara sauce
- One (1) slice mozzarella cheese
- Two (2) tbsp. pepperoni slices

Instructions:
1. Using a medium-high heat, heat oil in a skillet. Use salt and pepper to season the chicken.
2. Combine the seasoned chicken and garlic to skillet. Cook chicken until browned.
3. Tip in the pizza or marinara sauce on top. Let it simmer until sauce is heated.
4. Use a slice of mozzarella cheese and pieces of pepperoni to top each piece of chicken.
5. Cover the skillet until cheese is melted or put the skillet under the broiler to melt cheese.

(Calories: 337, fat: 18g, total carbs: 3g, net carbs: 2g, protein: 37g.)
Cabbage

Jamaican Jerk Pork Roast

Nutrition Info:

Calories, 240

Fat; 11g

(2 g saturated) fat

Sodium; 510 mg

Ingredients:

- 1 1/2 teaspoons ground allspice
- 1 1/2 teaspoons salt
- 1/2 teaspoon ground black pepper
- 1/2 teaspoon ground thyme
- 1/2 teaspoon ground cinnamon
- 1/4 teaspoon ground nutmeg
- 1/8 teaspoon ground cloves
- 3 green onions, chopped
- cloves garlic, minced
- 2 jalapeno
- 1 medium onion, chopped
- 1 lemon, juice
- 3 teaspoons oil
- 2 teaspoons soy sauce
- 2 teaspoons malt vinegar

- 1 teaspoon minced ginger root
- 3-4 lbs. cubed pork butt (2 inch chunks)

Directions:

1. In a large bowl combine the first 7 ingredients.
2. Mix thoroughly.
3. In a food processor combine green onions and garlic, pepper, onion, lemon juice, oil, soy sauce, malt vinegar and ginger.
4. Blend until very smooth.
5. Place pork in a glass bowl or large freezer bag, combine all ingredients and coat pork well.
6. Cover and stir or flip often.
7. Marinate for at least 8 hours.
8. Take out of the fridge 1 hour before grilling.
9. Preheat grill to medium high, skewer pork, 4 cubes to a skewer.
10. Cook for 6-8 minutes on one side, flip and 6-8 minutes on the other.

Zuppa Toscana

Nutrition Info:

Calories; 554

Fat; 32.6 g

Carbohydrates; 45.8 g

Protein; 19.8 g

Cholesterol, 99 mg

Ingredients:

- 1 pound bulk mild Italian sausage
- 1 1/4 teaspoons crushed red pepper flakes
- 4 slices bacon, cut into 1/2 inch pieces
- 1 large onion, diced
- 1 tablespoon minced garlic
- 5 (13.75 ounce) cans chicken broth
- 6 potatoes, thinly sliced1 cup heavy cream
- 1/4 bunch fresh spinach, tough stems removed.

Directions:

1. Cook the Italian sausage and red pepper flakes in a Dutch oven over medium-high heat until crumbly, browned, and no

longer pink, 10 to 15 minutes. Drain and set aside.

2. Cook bacon in the same Dutch oven over medium heat until crisp, about 10 minutes. Drain, leaving a few tablespoons of drippings with the bacon in the bottom of the Dutch oven. Stir in the onions and garlic; cook until onions are soft and translucent, about 5 minutes.
3. Pour chicken broth into the Dutch oven with the bacon and onion mixture; bring to a boil over high heat. Add potatoes, and boil until fork tender, about 20 minutes.
4. Reduce the heat to medium and stir in the heavy cream and cooked sausage, heat through.
5. Mix the spinach into the soup just before serving.

Thai Shrimp Soup.

Nutrition Info:

Calories; 368

Fat; 32.9 g

Carbohydrates; 8.9 g

Protein; 13.2 g

Cholesterol; 86 mg

Sodium; 579 mg

Ingredients:

- 1 tablespoon vegetable oil
- 2 tablespoons grated fresh ginger
- 1 stalk lemongrass, minced
- 2 teaspoons red curry paste
- 4 cups chicken broth
- 3 tablespoons fish sauce
- tablespoons fish sauce
- 1 tablespoon light brown sugar
- 3 (13.5 ounce) cans coconut milk
- 1/2 pound fresh shiitake mushrooms, sliced
- 1 pound medium shrimp - peeled and deveined
- 2 tablespoons fresh lime juice salt to taste
- 1/4 cup chopped fresh cilantro.

Directions:

1. Heat the oil in a large pot over medium heat. Cook and stir the ginger, lemongrass, and curry paste in the heated oil for 1 minutes.
2. Slowly pour chicken broth over the mixture, stirring continually. Stir in the fish sauce and brown sugar; simmer for 15 minutes. Stir in coconut milk and mushrooms;
3. Cook and stir until the mushrooms are soft, about 5 minutes.
4. Add shrimp; cook until no longer translucent, about 5 minutes.
5. Stir in the lime juice; season with salt; garnish with cilantro.

Dessert:

Chocolate Avocado Ice Cream

Nutrition Info:

Calories 323

Fat 32g49%

Saturated Fat 16.4g103%

Cholesterol 41mg 14%

Sodium 21mg 1%

Potassium 613mg 18%

Carbohydrates 12.3g 4%

Fiber 7.4g 31%

Sugar 1.5g 2%

Protein 3.9g 8%

Ingredients:

- 2 avocados ripe and stoned
- 1/2 cup cacao powder
- 3/4 cup heavy/double cream
- 3/4 cup coconut milk from a can
- 1/2 cup powdered sweetener
- optional: cocoa nibs

Directions:

1. Place all ingredients in a food processor or mix with a hand blender until smooth.
2. Check and adjust sweetener if necessary.
3. Stir in the cocoa nibs, if using.
4. Place in a container lined with baking paper.

5. Cover and freeze for 4-6 hours. If frozen overnight, you'll have to let the ice-cream defrost for 20 minutes before attempting to scoop.

Mocha Mouse.

Ingredients Info:

Calories 130

Total Fat 1.5g 2%

Saturated Fat 1.5g 8%

Trans Fat 0g

Cholesterol 0mg

Sodium 310mg 13%

Total Carbohydrates 29g 11%

Dietary Fibers 1g 4%

Sugars 18g 36%

Protein 3g 6g.

Ingredients:
- 1-1/2 cups cold fat-free milk
- 1 Tbsp. Instant Coffee
- 1 pkg. (3.9 oz.) Chocolate Flavor Instant Pudding

- 1/4 tsp. ground cinnamon
- 2 cups thawed cool whip free
- Whipped Topping, divided

Directions:

1. Pour milk into medium bowl. Add coffee granules. Beat with whisk 2 min. Add dry pudding mix and cinnamon; beat 2 min. Stir in 1-1/2 cups cool whips.
2. Pour into individual dessert dishes.
3. Refrigerate 1 hour. Top with remaining cool whip just before serving.

Strawberry Rhubarb Custard

Nutrition Info:

Calories; 342

Fat; 11.1g

Carbohydrates; 57.4g

Protein; 4.8 g

Cholesterol; 74 mg

Sodium. 159 mg

Ingredients:

- 1 (9 inch) unbaked pie crust
- 3 cups rhubarb, sliced 1/4-inch thick
- 1 cup fresh strawberries, quartered
- 3 large eggs
- 1 1/2 cups white sugar
- 3 tablespoons milk
- 3 tablespoons all-purpose flour
- 1/4 teaspoon freshly grated nutmeg
- 1 tablespoon butter, diced
- 2 tablespoons strawberry jam
- 1/4 teaspoon.

Directions:

1. Preheat oven to 350 degrees F (175 degrees C). Place rolled-out pie crust in a 9-inch pie plate and set on a baking sheet lined with parchment paper or a silicone baking mat.
2. Combine rhubarb and strawberries in a bowl; transfer to the pie crust, distributing evenly.
3. Whisk eggs, sugar, milk, flour, and nutmeg together in a medium bowl.

4. Slowly pour filling over rhubarb mixture until it just reaches the top edge of the crust. Scatter diced butter evenly over the top of the filling. Lightly tap and shake the baking sheet to remove any air bubbles.
5. Transfer pie to the preheated oven and bake, turning halfway through, until rhubarb is tender and custard is set, about 1 hour.
6. Mix strawberry jam and water in a small bowl; heat in the microwave until warm, about 15 seconds. Glaze the top of the pie with the jam mixture and let cool. Refrigerate until ready to serve.

Crème Brulee

Nutrition Info:

Calories; 561

Fat; 50.1 g

Carbohydrates; 24.g

Protein; 5.8 g

Cholesterol; 417 mg

Sodium 55 mg

Ingredients:
- 6 egg yolks
- 6 tablespoons white sugar, divided
- 1/2 teaspoon vanilla extract
- 2 1/2 cups heavy cream
- 2 tablespoons brown sugar.

Directions:
1. Preheat oven to 300 degrees F (150 degrees C).
2. Beat egg yolks, 4 tablespoons white sugar and vanilla extract in a mixing bowl until thick and creamy.
3. Pour cream into a saucepan and stir over low heat until it almost comes to boil. Remove the cream from heat immediately. Stir cream into the egg yolk mixture; beat until combined.
4. Pour cream mixture into the top pan of a double boiler.

5. Stir over simmering water until mixture lightly coats the back of a spoon, about 3 minutes. Remove mixture from heat immediately and pour into a shallow heat-proof dish.
6. Bake in preheated oven for 30 minutes.
7. Remove from oven and cool to room temperature. Refrigerate for at least 1 hour or overnight.
8. Preheat oven to broil.
9. In a small bowl combine remaining 2 tablespoons white sugar and brown sugar. Sift this mixture evenly over custard. Place dish under broiler until sugar melts, about 2 minutes. Watch carefully so as not to burn.
10. Remove from heat and allow to cool. Refrigerate until custard is set again.

Pumpkin Pie Pudding.

Nutrition Info:

Calories, 229

Fat; 9g

(5g saturated fat),

Cholesterol, 76mg

Sodium; 187 mg

Carbohydrates; 33g

(25g sugars, 2g fiber),

protein.6g

Ingredients:

- 1 can (15 ounces) solid-pack pumpkin
- 1 can (12 ounces) evaporated milk
- 3/4 cup sugar
- 1/2 cup biscuit/baking mix
- 2 large eggs, beaten
- 2 tablespoons butter, melted
- 2-1/2 teaspoons pumpkin pie spice
- 2 teaspoons vanilla extract
- Sweetened whipped cream or vanilla ice cream, optional

Directions:

1. Combine first eight ingredients. Transfer to a greased 3-qt. slow cooker.

2. Cook, covered, on low until a thermometer reads 160°, 6-7 hours. If desired.
3. Serve with whipped cream.

Thank you for purchasing our guide!

Made in the USA
Monee, IL
08 July 2022